Running: Your Fir

A beginner's guide to running

Table of Contents:

Introduction:

I am a middle distance athlete and runner who had found success using the tips that I am going to share with you in this E-book. I have won cross-country races through my earlier teenage years and placed well in other competitive track events. My aim throughout this guide is to help those who have not started the sport of running, or cycling or weightlifting to be able to start their fitness journey and to help those who are already there to become better athletes.

Now while to some, running may sound great and to others it may sound like a horror, there is a far cry between accomplishing the feat of running your first mile and what has been described on the previous page. Many people new to running fear it, but through this book, I am going to show you how to embrace it and how to start *your first mile.*

So as you read this book, always consult your doctor and a fitness professional before you do anything that has been mentioned. Do remember that you should take your first steps into fitness at your own pace and that you will become good, it just takes time. I hope that you enjoy!

Thank you for reading this book and I hope that you enjoy it!

Chapter 1: Preparing for the run

Contrary to popular belief; running for me has always been 80% mental strength and 20% physical. I see it this way as before running become even more natural to you than it already is to your body (Running is the most natural movement that the body can perform. E.g. a human babies cycle of crawling, learning to walk, then learning to run), you have to think about the run and where you will run to.

Other questions are how long will you run for? These questions soon add up and before you know it, the process has ended before it's started because you have given up and told yourself that it's a waste of time.

Here are a few tips that I used eight years ago when I started to take running seriously.

Do not concentrate on the length of the run:

If you are planning to go for your first run or a warm-up run for the more intermediate and advanced runners out there, focus on your first few steps. It may sound simple or patronising but if you let your feet perform the small steps of walking and then building into a small run, you are on your way.

When you concentrate on the length of the run, you can allow yourself to become intimidated by the very thought of running. It becomes hard and scary and all of a sudden you find yourself back in front of the tv on the sofa/couch watching the same old reality tv show kicking yourself at the fact that you didn't exercise today. DO NOT worry about the length of the run, just start and you can build your run over time. I'll touch on this a little later on in the book.

Allow yourself to clear your mind:

A lot of people like to listen to music when they run and that's not necessarily a bad thing. Playing music through earphones/headphones often allows you to get carried away in the run, often trying to match the rhythm of your feet with the music. However having earphones in can also provide distractions for 'newbies' and more experienced runners alike.

Earphones can often fall out whilst running which has caused me personally on more than one occasion to break my stride. They are also potential hazards, especially if like a lot of other runners; you are running in a city environment with constant traffic and driveways with reversing cars. These cars are often not seen or heard due to earphones being plugged in and played loudly and can be hazardous. (This applies to cyclists as well, even more so.)

Lastly earphones and listening to music/podcasts can take you away from the very experience of running. Whether running for pleasure, competition or relaxation, the essence of running is running whilst experiencing your surroundings. Akin to cycling and other endurance sports, your surroundings affect your ability to dominate your sport. So if the scenery is not great, you may be forgiven for running with earphones, but if you can, run without them as I find that it has allowed me to experience the nature of the run in its purest form.

By finding your moment of clarity whilst running or training, I have found that I actually enjoyed it a lot more. It was not a chore, I didn't have to hype myself up to exercise and I ended up being quite productive. That's not to say that you cannot exercise with music or podcasts because you can be very successful when doing so, but try doing without it at the start and see how you feel.

Chapter 2: The stretch

Many cardiovascular and strength athletes alike do not stretch when beginning to train and I used to be one of these athletes. Starting from cold would be the best way to run I thought.

However, the best way to prevent injury whilst running your first mile is to use a system called dynamic stretching.

Dynamic stretching is a method of stretching which allows the body to be warmed up correctly for the activity that will be performed, without limiting the body's ability to function.

This includes:

- **'The Axis'**- Balance on one leg, and whilst doing so, lift your other leg and bend it at a 90 degree angle sideways and hold this foot with your opposite hand. (Hold this position for 5 seconds and then release). <- Repeat this position with your alternate position.

This stretch can be repeated up to four times.

What does it stretch? =It stretches the hips and the thighs, preventing soreness and cramping.

- **'Open Gates'**- Lifting your knee (left or right) to chest height, you then slowly move your knee away to the right of your body whilst keeping it in mid-air. Lower the position once the knee has been extended away from the body. You can lower your knee away from your body at a rate of 2-3 seconds.

This stretch can be repeated as many times as you feel necessary

What does it stretch? = This stretches your hips and prevents tightness in your ability to move your hips freely.

- **'High Knees'** –This is a relatively simple stretch which allows the runner (you) to bring your knees up to your chest one knee at a high time. This is done whilst either jogging in one position or jogging slowly for the more intermediate/advanced runners.

This stretch can be repeated up to twenty times, hold the position and then repeat with alternate leg

What does this stretch? =This stretches the groin without placing unnecessary pressure on the groin and your knees.

- **'Sides to sides'** – This stretch which sees the athlete (you) move sideways (Can move arms up and down your sides whilst doing the initial stretch. Whilst moving sideways, the runner is running at a slow moderate pace. This stretch allows the runner to gently warm their calf muscles and also to get the body used to the motion of running.

This stretch can be performed up to ten times on each side

(Suggestion: This dynamic stretch should be performed at the start of exercising in order to gently warm the muscles preparing for the training ahead.)

- **'Calf Raises'** – This is a dynamic stretch that I like to perform at the start of my runs and also at the end of my training sessions as a method of cooling the body down.

For this stretch, you will need to find a set of stairs or a wall. You have to place both feet on the stairs and then lift yourself into the air with your calf muscles, pause for 2 seconds and then lower yourself down to the count of 3 seconds.

This stretch can be performed up to eight times and not only stretches the gastrocnemius 'big head' calf muscle, but also primes the muscle for tension, ready the body for muscle growth and full sporting activity such as running.

Summary:

Stretching is essential to any person who is training. It allows you not only to prevent injury but it also increases flexibility. It is a must for any training session and it's one element that is always needed within any sporting/training environment.

Chapter 3: The Warm Up Run:

The warm up run to me is essential to your first mile. Without a warm up run, you are much more prone to injury as your muscles are 'cold' before exercise. 'Cold muscles' meaning that the muscles had not had the opportunity to become used to the activity (the run) that is about to take place.

The warm up run that I would recommend to a beginner consists of; a gentle walk with small strides for about a minute. After the small strides for approximately one minute, I then would recommend moving into a small jog with moderate steps that are comfortable for you.

This light jog does not have to be a full jog/jog progression into a run. Instead I have personally jogged lightly for ten seconds and then stopped. This process would be repeated around four times in order to allow your legs to become acclimatised to the movement and to warm up properly.

If you combine this gentle warm-up run with the dynamic stretching that was described before, you will definitely be prepared to take on your first mile.

It's also important to note that if you are a complete beginner to running then you do not need to do everything at once. By this I mean you do not have to do a full run straight away. You can start with a warm up run/jog.

In doing so, you will allow yourself the opportunity to gain confidence from beginning slowly and you will also prevent yourself from overworking. This is how I started out and it allowed me to build a solid foundation not just for running but for my fitness.

Summary:

-Warm up runs are essential

-Begin and don't look back.

Chapter 4: How long to train for

This chapter will seek to explain how long you will train for.

Ideally if you are new to running I believe that you should attempt to run for a period of three to five minutes. Now to some that may seem like there is not a point to running for five minutes. However, those five minutes allow you to become used to running. As your body has now warmed up and has become primed to run, starting to run for three to five minutes will allow you as the beginner to become used to the way in which you run and your stride length.

Stride Length:

Your stride can be the most important thing when you are running as it determines what pace you will be setting, the length of your run and also your body position when running. Your stride when running can prevent injury and can also determine your level of productivity.

So now that we have established why your stride is important, it is important to note what an accurate stride length for your body is. For me I feel that setting a '1-2' pace is the best pace for my body to have a good run. A '1-2' pace consists of starting on your dominant leg with the count of 1 and then your secondary leg on the count of two. I start counting the 1-2 pace and continue to count until this pace becomes natural to my body. When this happens, I then start to increase my pace but keep my stride length consistent.

A consistent stride length not only allows for a steady, continuous pace, it also allows for greater balance. By your feet becoming aligned with each and moving together in tandem, you then find yourself being more balanced. I have found that a balanced upright position when running or jogging has allowed me to cover ground quickly and safely.

How long will my first run last?

This is a question that many newcomers and intermediate runners both ask? How long should my run last? What is the optimal time for a first jog or a 'normal run'?

In my opinion from experience there is no best length of time to start and complete a run. I personally started running by running to the end of my road from my house and then back again. I would repeat this cycle for as long as I had energy and then I would return and warm down. However, that was a bit different as I was ignoring the pain barrier and pushing myself into minor injuries that were unnecessary.

I then began to run up and down my road for two to three laps and then I began to branch out into the surrounding roads near to my house. I then progressed from there.

Building Blocks

So I do not believe that there is not a set correct length of time that you should be running for.

My method of running for two or three laps up and down my road will be of a benefit to the more intermediate runner the most; this is as they will be more used to running than the beginner. The beginner, could start running for a period of time by setting the end of a road as a benchmark.

This would allow the beginner runner/jogger to gather his/her stride and to increase the cardiovascular output. From this building block, beginners would be able to progress and become a 'cardiowarrior'.

Start at your own pace, build a little further every week and go from there. Your first mile is not a sprint, it's a marathon!

Chapter 5: How to improve your consistency:

Tip 1: Run Small

As I previously mentioned in the previous chapter, you do not need to put in long hours for your running and conditioning to improve. By running in small increments your fitness will improve allowing you to run for longer periods. However, running for longer periods takes time and the next tip will help with that.

Tip 2: Run Often

Just like anything in life, running requires practice. By running more your running will improve. Using a guide of running twice a week for 5-10 mins and then potentially increasing the volume to running twice a week for 10-20 minutes, this allows you to increase your workload whilst also increasing your distance/time.

This would progress to running three times a week for a period of 5-30 minutes each time.

Increasing the volume of running in the past allowed my body to become used to the demands of running and therefore preventing frequent injuries due to the motions that my body then became used to.

Tip 3: Allow your body to recover:

Now whilst the old saying of more is better is true. Doing more whilst remaining in great shape is critical for any person.

Resting the body and allowing the body to gain between 7-9 hours of sleep is crucial to allowing your body to recover, your muscles to repair and for a greater clarity of mind. Resting will allow you to attack the run or your training session with great energy the next day.

TAKE A BREAK

It may seem that I am stressing the importance of recovery but recovery is essential as your muscles repair themselves during periods of rest. I have personally found that my body responds well to three weeks of intense work (training) followed by 3-4 days of complete recovery.

There are fitness professionals and trainees who believe that when you are exercising or training that you should not take any days off. This philosophy is not an incorrect one. I am a firm believer in pushing the body to new levels of fitness.

However, it is VERY beneficial to allow for breaks between tough physical activity. The results in doing so from my experience? Greater energy supply; stronger muscles that have not suffered significant injury and increased muscle mass.

As a fitness athlete who focuses on running and weightlifting, I find this beneficial to my progress. I am not going to tell you fitness 'bro science', just what works for me as I believe that it can work for you too and allow you to be successful in your fitness journey.

Chapter 6: Exercises for Running

I recognise that taking the first of many steps in your fitness journey is an on-going process. It's not one that will be recognised straight away and it can be a difficult lifestyle to adapt to.

The following exercises are for the beginner, intermediate and advanced runner alike and they will help to strengthen and tone your body for exercise, especially running in this case.

-The Lunge:

I believe that the lunging motion which incorporates your hips, your knees and your lower back is vital to sustainability. This is because your hips need to be able to move and be flexible. Your knees whilst running are always moving so it is important to stretch them. Your lower back is very important and this cannot be stressed enough as when running, you can accidentally find yourself hunching over or arching.

The lunge is an exercise that can prevent you from arching as it keeps your back straight, allowing your body to become accustomed to the movement when moving.

-The push-up/press-up:

Now whilst the push-up is an exercise that is used primarily for upper body training and power related sports, I have found in my experience

that it is also useful for endurance athletes. This is as the push-up is an upper body compound movement.

By engaging the front, rear and side deltoids (shoulders) (depending on angle), trapezius (Traps), and chest, this exercise serves as a stability exercise that I use weekly to prevent injury. This is so that when I am running, my arms are always moving in conjunction with the rest of my upper body including my core (Abdominal muscles). This does not mean that injury will not occur, but I have prevented injury with this movement for many years.

-The squat:

Squatting is an exercise I use (twice a week) in order to improve my posture and in order to strengthen my quadriceps and hamstrings (Thigh muscles).

By squatting to varying degrees of height, my hips and my thighs just as in the lunge movement are engaged allowing the muscles to take on greater stress when running.

This will allow for greater power in your stride therefore allowing you to have a more efficient run. Squats are also a great fat burner as it is a full body movement, so for anybody wishing to burn fat this is an exercise to perform up to three times a week.

-Calf Raises:

Calf raises help to strengthen your ankles for the inevitable pressure that you place upon them when running. These raises can be done to the count of 3 or to the count of 5 depending upon how long you wish to hold it for.

Do not apply too much pressure as it can have an effect on your ankles

-The Plank:

Hold this position for 10 seconds at a time if you are a beginner to increase your core strength.

For intermediate/ advanced runner you could include the plank with an arm stretched out in front of the body. (This increases core stability and allows for greater balance.) I found this to be very helpful when running.

-The Kick-back:

Kick-backs are when you kick away from the body with one of your legs whilst either kneeling (in a plank position) or standing next to a flat surface and pushing away from it with one of your legs.

Your legs and your glutes are moving away from your body whilst your core is remaining firm throughout the exercise. This exercise not only strengthens the hamstrings but also adds definitive muscle tone. I personally noticed this whilst performing repetitions of 8-12 reps.

Summary:

These are the most basic exercises that you can add to your running routine in order to improve your conditioning and your posture. Other exercises that can be included are single-leg squats and pull-ups. Although these are exercises that seem basic, these have been the basis of my running routine and have kept me stable and strong for eight years.

Chapter 7: Best Foods:

Nutrition is a key part of health and wellness. Without it the body can become brittle and break down under the pressure of consistent exercise. Now although this book is an entry level guide to running and to exercising, it is very important to have key nutritious principles that you can follow.

So below I am going to outline the 10 best foods that I have found to be beneficial when I started to exercise regularly. These are below:

Almonds

A great source of protein which are essential to restoring the body after any form of exercise. Almonds are also high in fibre and have been known to help promote a healthy heart. They are a great healthy snack to have before bed. As for me I normally have these raw or place them into my porridge at the start of the day.

Blueberries

Blueberries are a natural anti-oxidant and are great at fighting off infections from the body. They are also a tasty way of getting fruit into the body and I often have these in my smoothies and in my porridge. Delicious and healthy.

Brown Rice

Brown rice is a whole grain and is rich in fibre. Great food for adding bulk whilst training and generally quite filling as opposed to white rice in my opinion.

Brown Pasta

Once again this is a whole grain that is rich in fibre and can be used as a good base for any meals that you have. It also contains carbohydrates which I found essential post training. It is quite tasty when mixed with a homemade tomato sauce and is very filling.

Quinoa

This is a grain that contains all 8 branch chain amino acids (BCAA's) which are essential nutrients that contribute to repairing muscle and keeping them healthy. It is a great source of protein and also contains nutrients that are useful in reducing inflammation in the body.

Kale

This is my favourite food out of everything mentioned. It is a great source of calcium and contains a high amount of vitamin A which essential for healthy eyesight and skin. This is more of a green that I love to have because it also fights inflammation which is essential to combat when training as it can cause irritation and pain. I have added Kale to various pasta sauces and dishes.

Bell Peppers

Bell peppers are great food for boosting and protecting the immune system. Found these to be extremely helpful when I started to train as I did not catch many colds when I started to include these in my diet.

Bananas

Bananas are great for anyone who trains as they contain vitamin C, vitamin B6 and potassium. A great source of energy post training session/ post workout and you can carry them anywhere in your gym bag/work bag.

Rye Bread

Rye bread is a bread that is quite light but full of fibre and nutrients which allows you to feel quite full without having to eat a lot of it. Very helpful for me when I was training for a run as I didn't want to eat a lot but have quite a bit of energy. Can often be found with seeds incorporated into them such as chia which are a great source of protein and fibre.

Flaxseeds

Flaxseeds are seeds that are high in fibre and also have a high amount of omega 3 fatty acids. These are great to have in your porridge before running in the morning or to have a snack in between meals. Once again essential due to the level of fibre and I did experience weight loss when using them regularly.

These are all foods that I have used consistently in my fitness journey. In fact, they even helped me to achieve a personal goal of running three times a day and staying injury free.

Conclusion:

So now I believe that you are primed to start your fitness journey. This short e-book was designed to help you as a runner, weightlifter, fitness athlete to become involved in running.

Running is not the only way to get started in your fitness journey but it is one of the best ways to begin as:

-YOU DO NOT NEED ANY EQUIPMENT.

-IT IS NOT TIME CONSUMING.

-IT IS FUN.

Most of all running is fun. It can be difficult, it can be challenging but knowing that there is nobody other than you on the road or on track who can push you to achieve your fitness goals, means that running will allow you to achieve your goals.

Running creates:

-Consistency

-Dedication (This is as sometimes during a run you will want to give up.)

-Achievement (This is as every run can be improved upon, whether that's your time, your stride or your overall general fitness.)

-Leaner look- For those looking to slim down and become leaner, I have found running to be my best and most consistent way to keep in 'lean state' all year around.

Hopefully, this book will allow you to get started in your running and your fitness journey and you can go on to achieve the level of fitness that you want.